2018
国际医学教育研究前沿报告

International Medical Education Research Fronts Reports

主编 闻德亮

科学出版社
北京

内 容 简 介

随着教育国际化不断发展，要求越来越多的医学院校和专家学者加强对医学教育发展的认识，及时更新国际先进教育教学理念。本报告通过文本挖掘的最新技术，全面梳理近10年国际医学教育目前的发展状态、识别医学教育研究领域最新的研究热点与方向，创新性地对目前纳入分析的2万余篇文献从"教育阶段""研究领域""临床医师岗位胜任力"三个维度进行标引分类，对纳入分类文献的高频主题词进行排序，发现毕业后教育、课程、教育技术、临床技能与医疗服务能力、核心价值观与医师职业精神成为热点关注的内容。通过引文共被引聚类分析总结归纳出七个研究热点与方向。通过这样的平台与数据信息，以期能够帮助全球的医学教育研究者、工作者紧跟时代步伐，共促医学教育的长足发展。

图书在版编目 (CIP) 数据

2018 国际医学教育研究前沿报告 / 闻德亮主编 . —北京：科学出版社，2018.7
ISBN 978-7-03-058322-2

Ⅰ.① 2… Ⅱ.①闻… Ⅲ.①医学教育－研究报告－世界－ 2018 Ⅳ.① R-4

中国版本图书馆 CIP 数据核字（2018）第 155747 号

责任编辑：王 颖／责任校对：郭瑞芝
责任印制：张欣秀／封面设计：王 融

科 学 出 版 社 出版
北京东黄城根北街 16 号
邮政编码：100717
http://www.sciencep.com
北京建宏印刷有限公司 印刷
科学出版社发行 各地新华书店经销

*

2018 年 7 月第 一 版 开本：720×1000 B5
2018 年 7 月第一次印刷 印张：3
字数：60 000
定价：19.80 元
（如有印装质量问题，我社负责调换）

《2018 国际医学教育研究前沿报告》
编写委员会

前　言

教育强国是中华民族伟大复兴的基础工程，人民健康是民族昌盛和国家富强的重要标志。党的十九大提出要优先发展教育事业，实施健康中国战略。因此，医学教育的改革发展承担着培养合格的卫生人才和提升全民健康的重任。为了在相互依存的世界里实现更好的医学教育，要求越来越多的医学院校和专家学者需要及时更新国际先进的教育教学理念，了解国际医学教育的现状和发展趋势，不断开拓医学教育研究与改革的新未来。

中国医科大学国际医学教育研究院前身为中国医科大学医学教育研究中心，自1981年成立至今，研究院经过30余年的探索与发展，逐步形成了借鉴国际先进医学教育理念和经验，结合中国国情进行研究实践，形成具有中国特色的医学教育改革和研究成果，并将成果推广应用的研究实践思路。中国医科大学国际医学教育研究院作为以"育人为本，国际视野，立足国情，服务社会"为使命的国际化医学教育研究机构，有责任也有义务向国家宏观决策层、专家学者和社会全面系统地报告国际医学教育研究的发展情况，这将有助于把握国际医学教育的整体发展态势和趋势，对未来发展进行前瞻性的思考和展望。

2018年，中国医科大学国际医学教育研究院通过文本挖掘的最新技术，全面梳理近10年国际医学教育目前的发展状态、识别医学教育研究领域最新的研究热点与方向发布了《2018国际医学教育研究前沿报告》。通过介绍医学教育研究的学术论文发表概况，如学科分布、国家分布和机构排名等，创新性地从"教育阶段""研究领域""临床医师岗位胜任力"三个维度概括医学教育研究的前沿进展，以期为专家学者的研究与医学院校的教育教学改革工作提供方向，为国家医学教育发展战略的制定和政策咨询提供参考，为国家宏观教育决策提供重要依据。

本研究报告的发布离不开科睿唯安团队的通力合作与科学出版社的大力

支持。我们在编写过程中力争保证资料的全面性和准确性。参与该项目的专家学者们开展了一系列的研讨会、审稿会等过程，将撰写的每一个细节力争做到最好。但也由于时间、精力和编写能力有限，本研究报告中的问题和失当之处在所难免，恳切希望各位同道和读者批评指正。

闻德亮

2018 年 7 月 5 日

中国医科大学

目　　录

2018 国际医学教育研究前沿报告

背　景

教育强国是中华民族伟大复兴的基础工程，人民健康是民族昌盛和国家富强的重要标志。因此，医学教育的发展与改革承担着培养合格的医疗卫生人才和提升全民健康的重任。为了在相互依存的世界里实现更好的医学教育，要求越来越多的医学院校和专家学者需要及时更新国际先进的教育教学理念，了解国际医学教育的现状和发展趋势，不断开拓医学教育研究与改革的新未来。但是，面对这种高速发展，仍然缺乏通过文献数据信息追踪和发现研究前沿的范式探究。因此，我们有责任也有义务提供这样一个平台和数据信息，以期为专家学者的研究与医学院校的教学改革工作提供方向，为国家医学教育发展战略的制定和政策咨询提供参考，为国家宏观教育决策提供重要依据。

目　的

基于权威的数据库，全面梳理近 10 年全球医学教育目前的发展状态；通过文本挖掘的最新技术，识别医学教育研究领域最新的研究热点方向。因此，中国医科大学与科睿唯安合作，通过跟踪全球重要的科学和学术论义，发布一年一度的研究前沿报告。

方　法

一、数据采集分析

在 PubMed 的 Mesh 主题词进行检索，收集分类为 Medical Education 2008 ~ 2017 年文献 PMID 号。与科睿唯安公司的 Web of Science 数据库（均为 SCIE 或 SSCI 收录文章）进行匹配，下载包括参考文献在内的全记录题录。

二、文献概览分析

在第一步的数据集收集整理的基础上，基于 Web of Science 数据库文献题录的信息和分类，对如下指标进行统计分析，包括：发文趋势、发文量排名前十国家、发文量排名前十机构、重点学科及主要刊载的期刊。

三、研究前沿分析

1. 高频主题词分析

基于科睿唯安公司对医学教育相关研究论文的主题词与题目词条的抽取与合并结果，对出现的频次及对应文献记录数进行排序后，对文献记录数 10 次以上对应的词条从"教育阶段""研究领域"和"临床医师岗位胜任力"三个维度进行标引分类。进而将纳入各个分类的论文主题词与题目抽取合并得到词条进行排序，分析高频词条内容（图 1）。

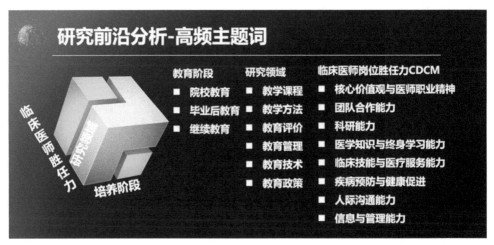

图 1　高频主题词分析

2. 引文共被引聚类分析

收集近 3 年（2015 ～ 2017）医学教育相关研究论文，基于中国医科大学崔雷教授开发的 Bicomb 软件对纳入本次分析的文献的引文进行抽取、排序及生成共被引矩阵，对被引频次在 100 次以上的引文使用 Gcluto 软件进行聚类分析（图 2）。

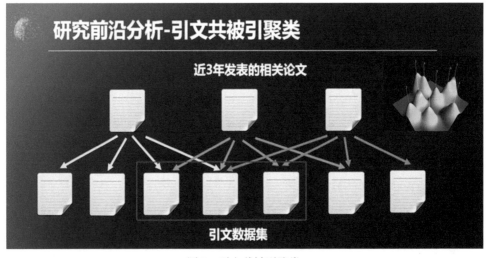

图 2　引文共被引聚类

结　果

一、文献概览

1. 发文趋势（图 3）

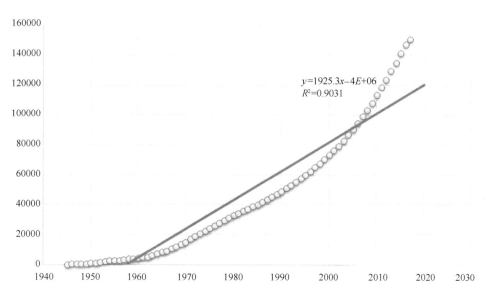

$$y=1925.3x-4E+06$$
$$R^2=0.9031$$

图 3　医学教育论文历史发文累计量

注：本次统计数据源为 1940 年以后发表的所有医学教育相关文献，检索策略为 Mesh 词：Education, Medical。

2. 国家分布（图 4）

序号	国家/地区	10年累计记录	百分比	序号	国家/地区	3年累计记录	百分比
1	USA	19798	51.584	1	USA	15185	51.565
2	ENGLAND	4113	10.717	2	ENGLAND	3219	10.931
3	CANADA	3643	9.492	3	CANADA	2825	9.593
4	AUSTRALIA	1994	5.195	4	AUSTRALIA	1544	5.243
5	GERMANY	1647	4.291	5	GERMANY	1208	4.102
6	NETHERLANDS	1229	3.202	6	NETHERLANDS	941	3.195
7	FRANCE	807	2.103	7	SCOTLAND	543	1.844
8	SCOTLAND	655	1.707	8	FRANCE	542	1.841
9	ITALY	542	1.412	9	INDIA	384	1.304
10	INDIA	483	1.258	10	ITALY	364	1.236
11	SPAIN	456	1.188	11	BRAZIL	337	1.144
12	SWITZERLAND	454	1.183	12	PEOPLES R CHINA	312	1.059
13	PEOPLES R CHINA	450	1.172	13	SPAIN	304	1.032
14	BRAZIL	433	1.128	14	SWITZERLAND	303	1.029
15	JAPAN	406	1.058	15	JAPAN	275	0.934

图 4　国家分布

3. 机构分布（图 5）

序号	机构	10年累计记录	百分比
1	HARVARD UNIVERSITY	2018	5.258
2	UNIVERSITY OF CALIFORNIA SYSTEM	1793	4.672
3	UNIVERSITY OF TORONTO	1296	3.377
4	VA BOSTON HEALTHCARE SYSTEM	1185	3.088
5	UNIVERSITY OF CALIFORNIA SAN FRANCISCO	873	2.275
6	UNIVERSITY OF TEXAS SYSTEM	818	2.131
7	MAYO CLINIC	808	2.105
8	UNIVERSITY OF PENNSYLVANIA	800	2.084
9	PENNSYLVANIA COMMONWEALTH SYSTEM OF HIGHER EDUCATION PCSHE	799	2.082
10	UNIVERSITY OF LONDON	781	2.035

序号	机构	3年累计记录	百分比
1	HARVARD UNIVERSITY	705	6.337
2	UNIVERSITY OF CALIFORNIA SYSTEM	586	5.267
3	UNIVERSITY OF TORONTO	419	3.766
4	VA BOSTON HEALTHCARE SYSTEM	418	3.757
5	UNIVERSITY OF PENNSYLVANIA	288	2.589
6	PENNSYLVANIA COMMONWEALTH SYSTEM OF HIGHER EDUCATION PCSHE	281	2.526
7	UNIVERSITY OF TEXAS SYSTEM	278	2.499
8	UNIVERSITY OF CALIFORNIA SAN FRANCISCO	276	2.481
9	UNIVERSITY OF MICHIGAN	253	2.274
10	UNIVERSITY OF MICHIGAN SYSTEM	253	2.274

图 5　机构分布

4. 学科分布（图 6）

序号	研究方向	10年累计记录	百分比
1	EDUCATION EDUCATIONAL RESEARCH	9983	26.011
2	HEALTH CARE SCIENCES SERVICES	8540	22.251
3	GENERAL INTERNAL MEDICINE	7463	19.445
4	SURGERY	6367	16.589
5	PEDIATRICS	1483	3.864
6	CARDIOVASCULAR SYSTEM CARDIOLOGY	1466	3.82
7	PUBLIC ENVIRONMENTAL OCCUPATIONAL HEALTH	1437	3.744
8	PSYCHIATRY	1415	3.687
9	RADIOLOGY NUCLEAR MEDICINE MEDICAL IMAGING	1346	3.507
10	NEUROSCIENCES NEUROLOGY	1135	2.957

序号	研究方向	3年累计记录	百分比
1	EDUCATION EDUCATIONAL RESEARCH	2845	25.573
2	HEALTH CARE SCIENCES SERVICES	2181	19.604
3	SURGERY	2059	18.508
4	GENERAL INTERNAL MEDICINE	2001	17.987
5	CARDIOVASCULAR SYSTEM CARDIOLOGY	478	4.297
6	RADIOLOGY NUCLEAR MEDICINE MEDICAL IMAGING	476	4.279
7	PSYCHIATRY	429	3.856
8	PEDIATRICS	414	3.721
9	PUBLIC ENVIRONMENTAL OCCUPATIONAL HEALTH	413	3.712
10	NEUROSCIENCES NEUROLOGY	323	2.903

图 6　学科分布

5. 期刊分布（图 7）

序号	来源出版物名称	10年累计记录	百分比
1	ACADEMIC MEDICINE	2143	5.584
2	MEDICAL EDUCATION	1786	4.653
3	MEDICAL TEACHER	1723	4.489
4	BMC MEDICAL EDUCATION	944	2.46
5	JOURNAL OF SURGICAL EDUCATION	871	2.269
6	ACADEMIC PSYCHIATRY	762	1.985
7	FAMILY MEDICINE	575	1.498
8	AMERICAN JOURNAL OF SURGERY	390	1.016
9	JOURNAL OF GENERAL INTERNAL MEDICINE	386	1.006
10	JAMA JOURNAL OF THE AMERICAN MEDICAL ASSOCIATION	376	0.98

序号	来源出版物名称	3年累计记录	百分比
1	ACADEMIC MEDICINE	592	5.321
2	MEDICAL EDUCATION	419	3.766
3	BMC MEDICAL EDUCATION	374	3.362
4	MEDICAL TEACHER	366	3.29
5	JOURNAL OF SURGICAL EDUCATION	322	2.894
6	ACADEMIC PSYCHIATRY	276	2.481
7	FAMILY MEDICINE	165	1.483
8	AMERICAN JOURNAL OF SURGERY	141	1.267
9	ADVANCES IN HEALTH SCIENCES EDUCATION	122	1.097
10	JOURNAL OF THE AMERICAN COLLEGE OF RADIOLOGY	114	1.025

图 7　期刊分布

二、研究前沿分析

1. 高频主题词分析

维度一

教育阶段：院校教育、毕业后教育、继续教育

2008 ~ 2017 年院校教育、毕业后教育和继续教育三类论文累计发文量分别为 4622、12627 和 3870。其中，毕业后教育相关论文发文量最大，尤其近 5 年来增长迅速（图 8）。

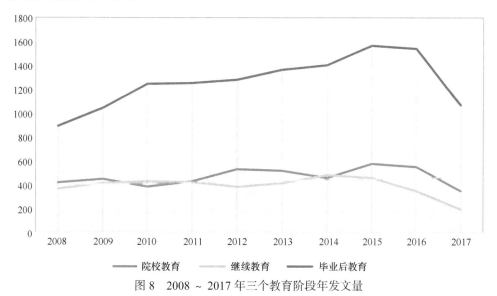

图 8　2008 ~ 2017 年三个教育阶段年发文量

注：2017 年 WOS 数据库从出版商出收录论文未完整，因此 2017 年度论文数不是最终数量，在 2019 年的研究前沿报告中，未包含的 2017 年部分文献将被纳入分析。

（1）院校教育

排名前 10 主题词

1）Curriculum

2）Simulation（近 3 年记录比率 46%）

3）Assessment

4）PBL

5）E-learning（近 3 年记录比率 48%）

6）Clinical skills

7）Communication skills

8）Professionalism

9）Career choice

10）Active learning

排名前 10 机构

1）Univ Toronto

2）Maastricht Univ

3）Univ Calif San Francisco

4）Harvard Univ

5）Univ Michigan（近 3 年记录比率 43%）

6）Monash Univ

7）Univ British Columbia

8）Univ Sydney

9）Univ Illinois（近 3 年记录比率 47%）

10）Univ Calgary

（2）毕业后教育

排名前 10 主题词

1）Simulation（近 3 年记录比率 44%）

2）Curriculum

3）Assessment

4）Patient safety

5）Communication skills

6）Teaching

7）Learning curve

8）Clinical competence

9）Primary care

10）Professionalism

排名前 10 机构

1）Harvard Univ

2）Univ Toronto

3）Univ Calif San Francisco

4）Mayo Clin

5）Univ Penn（近 3 年记录比率 40%）

6）Univ Michigan（近 3 年记录比率 39%）

7）Northwestern Univ

8）Univ Washington（近 3 年记录比率 41%）

9）Johns Hopkins Univ

10）Yale Univ

（3）继续教育

排名前 10 主题词

1）Primary care

2）Simulation（近 3 年记录比率 37%）

3）Quality Improvement

4）Assessment

5）Learning curve

6）E-learning

7）Palliative care（近 3 年记录比率 31%）

8）Teaching

9）Knowledge translation

10）Patient safety

排名前 10 机构

1）Univ Toronto

2）Harvard Univ

3）Mayo Clin

4）Univ Calif San Francisco

5）Univ Washington（近 3 年记录比率 38%）

6）McMaster Univ

7）Univ Ottawa（近 3 年记录比率 41%）

8）Univ Calgary（近 3 年记录比率 38%）

9）Johns Hopkins Univ

10）McGill Univ

维度二

研究领域：课程、教育技术、教育评价、教学方法、教育管理、教育政策

在医学教育研究领域中，关于课程及教育技术的相关论文发表量最大，超过纳入各个类别总量的一半以上（图 9）。

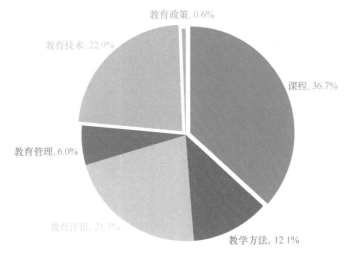

图 9　六类研究领域发文量分布

（1）课程

排名前 10 主题词

1）Competency-Based Education（近 3 年记录比率 38%）

2）Curriculum development

3）Milestones（近 3 年记录比率 70%）

4）Needs assessment

5）Feedback

6）Educational outcome

7）Simulation（近 3 年记录比率 57%）

8）Internship and residency

9）Learning（近 3 年记录比率 42%）

10）Pediatrics

排名前 10 机构

1）Univ Toronto（近 3 年记录比率 57%）

2）Harvard Univ（近 3 年记录比率 40%）

3）Univ Calif San Francisco（近 3 年记录比率 44%）

4）Yale Univ

5）Univ Massachusetts（近 3 年记录比率 71%）

6）Univ Ottawa（近 3 年记录比率 71%）

7）Univ Washington（近 3 年记录比率 57%）

8）Columbia Univ（近 3 年记录比率 67%）

9）Johns Hopkins Univ

10）Mayo Clin

（2）教育技术

排名前 10 主题词

1）Simulation（近 3 年记录比率 43%）

2）Training（近 3 年记录比率 41%）

3）E-learning

4）Virtual reality

5）Laparoscopy 腹腔镜检查

6）Surgical education（近 3 年记录比率 43%）

7）Internet

8）Assessment

9）Social media（近 3 年记录比率 67%）

10）Virtual patients（近 3 年记录比率 40%）

排名前 10 机构

1）Univ Toronto

2）Harvard Univ

3）Mayo Clin

4）Univ London Imperial Coll Sci Technol & Med

5）Northwestern Univ

6）McGill Univ（近 3 年记录比率 51%）

7）Univ Calgary

8）Univ Ottawa（近 3 年记录比率 52%）

9）Johns Hopkins Univ

10）NYU

（3）教育评价

排名前 10 主题词

1）Feedback（近 3 年记录比率 46%）

2）Training

3）Simulation（近 3 年记录比率 44%）

4）Certification

5）Needs assessment

6）Accreditation

7）Milestones（近 3 年记录比率 68%）

8）AMEE Guide

9）Program evaluation

10）OSCE

排名前 10 机构

1）Univ Toronto（近 3 年记录比率 38%）

2）Harvard Univ

3）Maastricht Univ

4）Univ Calif San Francisco（近 3 年记录比率 42%）

5）Mayo Clin

6）Univ Ottawa（近 3 年记录比率 52%）

7）Univ Calif Los Angeles

8）Univ Michigan（近 3 年记录比率 53%）

9）Univ Washington

10）Johns Hopkins Univ（近 3 年记录比率 39%）

（4）教学方法

排名前 10 主题词

1）Learning curve

2）Blended learning（近 3 年记录比率 42%）

3）Case study

4）Team-based learning

5）Simulation（近 3 年记录比率 56%）

6）E-learning

7）Experiential learning（近 3 年记录比率 47%）

8）Reflection

9）Standardized patients

10）Collaborative learning

排名前 10 机构

1）Maastricht Univ（近 3 年记录比率 46%）

2）Univ Toronto

3）Harvard Univ

4）Univ Calif San Francisco（近 3 年记录比率 39%）

5）Mayo Clin

6）Johns Hopkins Univ（近 3 年记录比率 54%）

7）Yale Univ（近 3 年记录比率 54%）

8）Brown Univ

9）Karolinska Inst

10）McGill Univ（近 3 年记录比率 70%）

（5）教育管理

排名前 10 主题词

1）Educational intervention（近 3 年记录比率 49%）

2）Workforce

3）Learning environment（近 3 年记录比率 40%）

4）School admission criteria（近 3 年记录比率 41%）

5）Specialty choice

6）Primary care

7）Educational impact

8）Continuing medical education（近 3 年记录比率 62%）

9）Educational needs/gaps

10）Guideline adherence

排名前 10 机构

1）Univ Toronto（近 3 年记录比率 67%）

2）Univ Michigan（近 3 年记录比率 73%）

3）Harvard Univ（近 3 年记录比率 50%）

4）Johns Hopkins Univ（近 3 年记录比率 60%）

5）Northwestern Univ（近 3 年记录比率 80%）

6）Mayo Clin

7）Univ Calif San Francisco

8）Univ N Carolina（近 3 年记录比率 44%）

9）Univ Washington

10）Univ Connecticut（近 3 年记录比率 62%）

（6）教育政策

排名前 10 主题词

1）Health services research

2）Rural health

3）Career choice

4）Career development

5）Emergency medicine

6）Family medicine

7）graduate medical education

8）Primary care

9）Quality of care

10）Workforce

排名前 10 机构

1）Robert Graham Ctr（近 3 年记录比率 60%）

2）Harvard Univ（近 3 年记录比率 67%）

3）Univ Calif Los Angeles

4）Univ Penn

5）Univ Toronto

6）Assoc Amer Med Coll（近 3 年记录比率 100%）

7）Dartmouth Coll（近 3 年记录比率 50%）

8）Jichi Med Univ

9）Univ Calif San Francisco

10）Univ Virginia（近 3 年记录比率 100%）

维度三

医师岗位胜任力：临床技能与医疗服务能力、核心价值观与医师职业精神、疾病预防与健康促进、科研能力、医学知识与终身学习能力、信息与管理能力、人际沟通能力、团队合作能力

在过去 10 年中，医师岗位胜任力各项发文量统计结果显示，临床技能与医疗服务能力、核心价值观与医师职业精神和疾病预防与健康促进方面的文量发表的最多，占总量的 75%（图 10）。

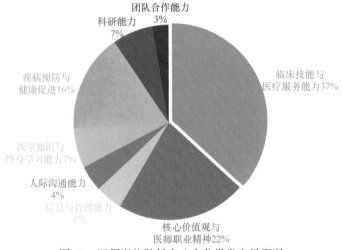

图 10　医师岗位胜任力八个分类发文量概况

（1）临床技能与医疗服务能力

排名前 10 主题词

1）Primary care

2）Patient safety（近 3 年记录比率 39%）

3）Simulation（近 3 年记录比率 40%）

4）Clinical reasoning（近 3 年记录比率 37%）

5）Quality Improvement

6）Quality assurance

7）Assessment

8）Diagnosis

9）Physical examination

10）End-of-life care

排名前 10 机构

1）Univ Toronto

2）Harvard Univ

3）Univ Calif San Francisco

4）Univ Washington

5）Mayo Clin

6）Maastricht Univ

7）Johns Hopkins Univ

8）Yale Univ

9）Univ Calgary

10）Univ Penn

（2）核心价值观与医师职业精神

排名前 10 主题词

1）Attitudes

2）Ethics（近 3 年记录比率 22%）

3）Workforce（近 3 年记录比率 32%）

4）Burnout（近 3 年记录比率 45%）

5）Empathy（近 3 年记录比率 43%）

6）Depression（近 3 年记录比率 39%）

7）Stress

8）Motivation（近 3 年记录比率 42%）

9）Training

10）Patient satisfaction

排名前 10 机构

1）Univ Toronto

2）Mayo Clin

3）Harvard Univ

4）Univ Calif San Francisco

5）Univ Michigan（近 3 年记录比率 52%）

6）Johns Hopkins Univ（近 3 年记录比率 41%）

7）Maastricht Univ（近 3 年记录比率 40%）

8）Massachusetts Gen Hosp（近 3 年记录比率 44%）

9）Univ Washington（近 3 年记录比率 44%）

10）Emory Univ（近 3 年记录比率 44%）

（3）疾病预防与健康促进

排名前 10 主题词

1）Quality improvement（近 3 年记录比率 47%）

2）Palliative care（近 3 年记录比率 39%）

3）Patient safety

4）Global health（近 3 年记录比率 49%）

5）Primary care

6）Curriculum（近 3 年记录比率 39%）

7）Graduate medical education（近 3 年记录比率 43%）

8）Older adults

9）Continuing medical education（近 3 年记录比率 48%）

10）Public health

排名前 10 机构

1）Univ Calif San Francisco（近 3 年记录比率 44%）

2）Harvard Univ

3）Univ Toronto（近 3 年记录比率 53%）

4）Univ Washington（近 3 年记录比率 63%）

5）Univ Calif Los Angeles（近 3 年记录比率 59%）

6）Johns Hopkins Univ（近 3 年记录比率 44%）

7）Univ Wisconsin

8）Emory Univ（近 3 年记录比率 43%）

9）Univ Michigan

10）Univ Minnesota（近 3 年记录比率 43%）

（4）科研能力

排名前 10 主题词

1）Academic performance

2）Basic science

3）Training

4）Clinical research

5）Academic Productivity（近 3 年记录比率 43%）

6）Critical thinking

7）Academic Detailing

8）Innovation（近 3 年记录比率 47%）

9）Curriculum

10）Problem solving

排名前 10 机构

1）Univ Toronto

2）Harvard Univ

3）Mayo Clin（近 3 年记录比率 45%）

4）Univ Calif San Francisco

5）Univ British Columbia

6）Univ Ottawa

7）Univ Pittsburgh

8）Yale Univ（近 3 年记录比率 50%）

9）McMaster Univ

10）Dalhousie Univ

（5）医学知识与终身学习能力

排名前 10 主题词

1）Self-directed learning（近 3 年记录比率 40%）

2）Active learning

3）Knowledge translation

4）Attitudes

5）Interdisciplinary communication（近 3 年记录比率 43%）

6）Assessment

7）Continuing medical education

8）Undergraduate medical education

9）Evidence-based medicine

10）PBL

排名前 10 机构

1）Univ Toronto

2）McMaster Univ（近 3 年记录比率 40%）

3）Univ Laval

4）Univ Calgary

5）Univ Alberta

6）Univ Michigan

7）Dalhousie Univ

8）Harvard Univ（近 3 年记录比率 50%）

9）Mayo Clin（近 3 年记录比率 62%）

10）St Michaels Hosp

（6）信息与管理能力

排名前 10 主题词

1）Leadership

2）Health Policy

3）Resident duty hours

4）Quality management

5）Medical informatics

6）Information technology

7）Health manpower

8）Patient safety

9）Risk management

10）Continuing medical education

排名前 10 机构

1）Harvard Univ（近 3 年记录比率 46%）

2）Univ Toronto

3）Baylor Coll Med（近 3 年记录比率 43%）

4）Mayo Clin（近 3 年记录比率 43%）

5）Yale Univ

6）Univ Calif Los Angeles

7）Univ Michigan

8）Univ Penn

9）Univ Washington

10）Emory Univ

（7）人际沟通能力

排名前 10 主题词

1）Assessment

2）Training

3）Interprofessional collaboration（近 3 年记录比率 44%）

4）Patient-physician relationship（近 3 年记录比率 47%）

5）OSCE（近 3 年记录比率 42%）

6）Professionalism

7）Simulation

8）Residents

9）Medical students

10）Breaking bad news

排名前 10 机构

1）Univ Toronto

2）Catholic Univ Louvain

3）Harvard Univ（近 3 年记录比率 38%）

4）Univ Libre Bruxelles

5）Univ Liege

6）Duke Univ（近 3 年记录比率 50%）

7）Monash Univ

8）Radboud Univ Nijmegen

9）Univ Calif San Francisco（近 3 年记录比率 60%）

10）Free Univ Brussels

（8）团队合作能力

排名前 10 主题词

1）Training

2）Simulation

3）Interprofessional education

4）Patient Safety

5）Leadership

6）Assessment

7）Surgery

8）Continuing medical education

9）Quality improvement

10）Faculty development

排名前 10 机构

1）Univ Toronto

2）Harvard Univ

3）Mayo Clin

4）Monash Univ

5）Univ Calif San Francisco（近 3 年记录比率 67%）

6）Univ London Imperial Coll Sci Technol & Med

7）Childrens Hosp Philadelphia

8）Karolinska Inst（近 3 年记录比率 50%）

9）Univ Sydney（近 3 年记录比率 50%）

10）Massachusetts Gen Hosp

注：在以上三个维度的 17 个分类中，surgical education 出现在多个分类的高频主题词中，结合医学教育相关学科及期刊发文量分布的结果，显示外科类教育的确在近年来日益受到关注，成为医学专科类别种医学教育研究最为重要的主战场。

2. 引文共被引聚类分析（图 11）

通过引文共被引聚类分析，近 3 年论文的高频引文的高频引文被聚类为以下七个主要方面：

（1）胜任力在医学教育中理论与实践。

（2）以能力为导向的评价及评价方法的研究。

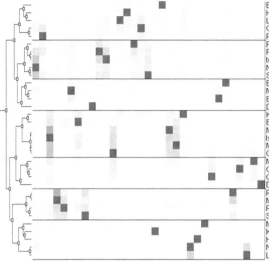

Braun V, 2006, QUALITATIVE RES PSYC, V3, P77
Hafferty FW, 1998, ACAD MED, V73, P403
Lave J, 1991, SITUATED LEARNING LE
Cooke M, 2010, ED PHYS CALL REFORM
Frenk J, 2010, LANCET, V376, P1923
Frank JR, 2005, CANMEDS 2005 PHYS CO
Frank JR, 2010, MED TEACH, V32, P638
ten Cate O, 2007, ACAD MED, V82, P542
Nasca TJ, 2012, NEW ENGL J MED, V366, P1051
Swing SR, 2007, MED TEACH, V29, P648
Epstein RM, 2002, JAMA-J AM MED ASSOC, V287, P2
MILLER GE, 1990, ACAD MED, V65, pS63
Epstein RM, 2007, NEW ENGL J MED, V356, P387
Davis DA, 2006, JAMA-J AM MED ASSOC, V296, P109
Kolb D., 1984, EXPERIENTIAL LEARNIN
Ericsson KA, 2004, ACAD MED, V79, pS70
McGaghie WC, 2010, MED EDUC, V44, P50
Issenberg SB, 2005, MED TEACH, V27, P10
McGaghie WC, 2011, ACAD MED, V86, P706
Cook DA, 2011, JAMA-J AM MED ASSOC, V306, P978
Moher D, 2009, BMJ-BRIT MED J, V339
Cook DA, 2008, JAMA-J AM MED ASSOC, V300, P118
Cohen J, 1988, STAT POWER ANAL BEHA
Davis D, 1999, JAMA-J AM MED ASSOC, V282, P867
Reznick R, 1997, AM J SURG, V173, P226
Martin JA, 1997, BRIT J SURG, V84, P273
Reznick RK, 2006, NEW ENGL J MED, V355, P2664
Seymour NE, 2002, ANN SURG, V236, P458
Mattar SG, 2013, ANN SURG, V258, P440
Kohn LT, 2000, ERR IS HUMAN BUILDIN
Harris PA, 2009, J BIOMED INFORM, V42, P377
Nasca TJ, 2010, NEW ENGL J MED, V363
Landrigan CP, 2004, NEW ENGL J MED, V351, P1838

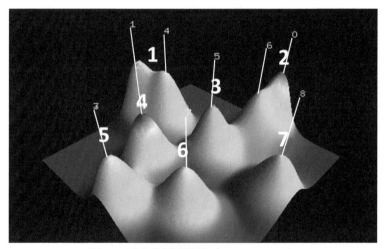

图 11　引文共被引聚类（2015 ~ 2017）

（3）模拟增强技术在医学教育学习和评价中的应用。

（4）临床实践能力的教学与评价。

（5）执业环境对住院医师和实习医学生学习和表现的影响。

（6）医学教育干预研究及干预效果评价。

（7）其他，包括学习环境、隐性课程等。

结　　论

1. 在国家累计发文量统计中，巴西与中国进步明显。

2. 在机构累计发文量统计中，宾夕法尼亚大学及其附属机构，近 3 年来增长显著。

3. 在学科累计发文量统计中，医学教育在外科学、心血管系统、精神疾病等方面近 3 年出现了更多的跨学科研究成果。

4. 在期刊累计发文量统计中，近 3 年新出现了 ADVANCES IN HEALTH SCIENCES EDUCATION 和 JOURNAL OF THE AMERICAN COLLEGE OF RADIOLOGY 位于发文量前 10 的期刊中。

5. 在三个维度中，毕业后教育、课程和教育技术、临床能力与医疗服务能力、核心价值观与医师职业精神成为热点关注的内容。

6. 教育阶段研究前沿分析中，主题词 Simulation，Primary care, Professionalism 和 Patient safety 在不同教育阶段中成为共同的关注热点。

7. 在医师岗位胜任力研究前沿分析中，核心价值观与医师职业精神，疾病预防与健康促进两个主题中，近 3 年出现频次增长较快的高频主题词过半，表明该两个研究主题近期受到更多关注。

8. 在研究领域前沿分析中，milestones 的培育理念和 social media 是近 3 年最为活跃的关注热点。 而 competency 及其相关词汇在多个研究领域高频主题词中均有出现。

9. 在引文共被引聚类分析中，除了胜任力在医学教育中的理论与实践、模拟增强技术的应用等聚类主题进一步印证了高频主题词的分析结果，仍有学习环境、隐性课程等内容在该分析中出现。

局限性

无论是高频主题词统计还是引文共被引聚类分析技术，均基于高频和高被引的数据指标，长于抓住重点而非覆盖全面。但是，在本研究中也通过三个维度的标引分类及分析，力争能够完整地描述整个医学教育研究版图。

致　谢

科睿唯安团队

2018 International Medical Education Research Fronts Report

Background

More and more universities and experts focus on the medical education research, and they all hope to explore the hot research topic through literature and practical experience. In addition, the pace of internationalization of medical education has increasingly become faster, which needs us to strengthen mutual understanding and updates our ideas timely. However, being faced with the rapid development, we still lack the paradigm research of taking advantage of literature to track the front research. Thus, we have the responsibility and mission to provide a platform and data to help the international researchers keep pace with the times and the world's development.

Objectives

（1）Based on authoritative database, review the development of international medical education in last 10 years.

（2）Based on the latest technology of text mining, recognize the hot research topic in the field of medical education research.

Thus, China Medical University collaborated with Clarivate to release the annual cutting-edge repot by tracking the global academic literature published in WOS database.

Methods

I. Data Collection

（1）Search the keyword "Mesh" on Pub Med and collect the PMID of the literature（2008-2017）which belong to "Medical Education".

（2）Matched the PMID with the literature in WOS database（including SCIE and SSCI）, and downloaded the whole literature including Reference.

II. Overview Analysis of Literature

After data collection, and based on the content and categories of WOS database about the country, publication year, institution and discipline, we analyzed the following index: Publication trend, Top countries, Top institutions and Top disciplines.

III. Research Fronts Analysis

1. High Frequent Keywords Analysis

Depending on the extracting item from the keywords and title of the medical education publication by the Clarivate group, we ranked the items by the appearance frequency in the publications. Then, we classified the items with appearance frequency in the publications more than 10 times by three domains（education phase, Research field, and Clinical physician competency）. Finally, we ranked the items from the publication that corresponded to the high frequency item in last ranking round and analyzed the content（Figure 1）.

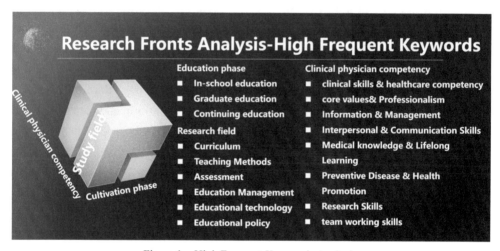

Figure 1   High Frequent Keywords Analysis

2. Reference Co-cited Clustering Analysis

We collected the medical education publications over the past three years（2015-2017）and extracted the citation, ranked them and developed the item-publication matrix by the Bicomb software. Then we clustered the citations that were cited more than 100 times by the Gcluto software（Figure 2）.

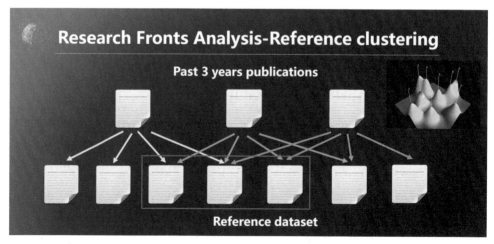

Figure 2   Reference Co-cited Clustering Analysis

Results

I. Overview

1. Trends of Publications（Figure 3）

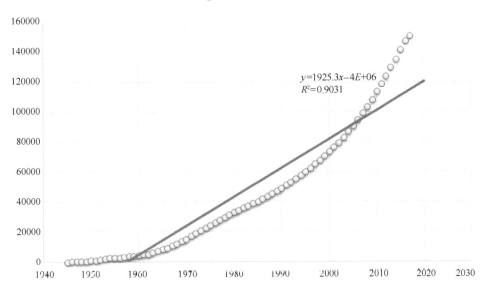

$$y=1925.3x-4E+06$$
$$R^2=0.9031$$

Figure 3　Accumulative Number of Publications

Note：The database for this analysis included the medical education publications from 1940 till now.

The Search strategy is Education, Medical [Mesh].

2. Distribution by Countries（Figure 4）

No.	Country	10 years number	Percentage	No.	Country	3 years number	Percentage
1	USA	19798	51.584	1	USA	15185	51.565
2	ENGLAND	4113	10.717	2	ENGLAND	3219	10.931
3	CANADA	3643	9.492	3	CANADA	2825	9.593
4	AUSTRALIA	1994	5.195	4	AUSTRALIA	1544	5.243
5	GERMANY	1647	4.291	5	GERMANY	1208	4.102
6	NETHERLANDS	1229	3.202	6	NETHERLANDS	941	3.195
7	FRANCE	807	2.103	7	SCOTLAND	543	1.844
8	SCOTLAND	655	1.707	8	FRANCE	542	1.841
9	ITALY	542	1.412	9	INDIA	384	1.304
10	INDIA	483	1.258	10	ITALY	364	1.236
11	SPAIN	456	1.188	11	BRAZIL	337	1.144
12	SWITZERLAND	454	1.183	12	PEOPLES R CHINA	312	1.059
13	PEOPLES R CHINA	450	1.172	13	SPAIN	304	1.032
14	BRAZIL	433	1.128	14	SWITZERLAND	303	1.029
15	JAPAN	406	1.058	15	JAPAN	275	0.934

Figure 4　Distribution in Countries

3. Distribution by Institutions (Figure 5)

No.	Institution	10 years number	Percentage	No.	Institution	3 years number	Percentage
1	HARVARD UNIVERSITY	2018	5.258	1	HARVARD UNIVERSITY	705	6.337
2	UNIVERSITY OF CALIFORNIA SYSTEM	1793	4.672	2	UNIVERSITY OF CALIFORNIA SYSTEM	586	5.267
3	UNIVERSITY OF TORONTO	1296	3.377	3	UNIVERSITY OF TORONTO	419	3.766
4	VA BOSTON HEALTHCARE SYSTEM	1185	3.088	4	VA BOSTON HEALTHCARE SYSTEM	418	3.757
5	UNIVERSITY OF CALIFORNIA SAN FRANCISCO	873	2.275	5	UNIVERSITY OF PENNSYLVANIA	288	2.589
6	UNIVERSITY OF TEXAS SYSTEM	818	2.131	6	PENNSYLVANIA COMMONWEALTH SYSTEM OF HIGHER EDUCATION PCSHE	281	2.526
7	MAYO CLINIC	808	2.105	7	UNIVERSITY OF TEXAS SYSTEM	278	2.499
8	UNIVERSITY OF PENNSYLVANIA	800	2.084	8	UNIVERSITY OF CALIFORNIA SAN FRANCISCO	276	2.481
9	PENNSYLVANIA COMMONWEALTH SYSTEM OF HIGHER EDUCATION PCSHE	799	2.082	9	UNIVERSITY OF MICHIGAN	253	2.274
10	UNIVERSITY OF LONDON	781	2.035	10	UNIVERSITY OF MICHIGAN SYSTEM	253	2.274

Figure 5　Distribution in Institutions

4. Distribution by Disciplines (Figure 6)

No.	Discipline	10 years number	Percentage	No.	Discipline	3 years number	Percentage
1	EDUCATION EDUCATIONAL RESEARCH	9983	26.011	1	EDUCATION EDUCATIONAL RESEARCH	2845	25.573
2	HEALTH CARE SCIENCES SERVICES	8540	22.251	2	HEALTH CARE SCIENCES SERVICES	2181	19.604
3	GENERAL INTERNAL MEDICINE	7463	19.445	3	SURGERY	2059	18.508
4	SURGERY	6367	16.589	4	GENERAL INTERNAL MEDICINE	2001	17.987
5	PEDIATRICS	1483	3.864	5	CARDIOVASCULAR SYSTEM CARDIOLOGY	478	4.297
6	CARDIOVASCULAR SYSTEM CARDIOLOGY	1466	3.82	6	RADIOLOGY NUCLEAR MEDICINE MEDICAL IMAGING	476	4.279
7	PUBLIC ENVIRONMENTAL OCCUPATIONAL HEALTH	1437	3.744	7	PSYCHIATRY	429	3.856
8	PSYCHIATRY	1415	3.687	8	PEDIATRICS	414	3.721
9	RADIOLOGY NUCLEAR MEDICINE MEDICAL IMAGING	1346	3.507	9	PUBLIC ENVIRONMENTAL OCCUPATIONAL HEALTH	413	3.712
10	NEUROSCIENCES NEUROLOGY	1135	2.957	10	NEUROSCIENCES NEUROLOGY	323	2.903

Figure 6　Distribution in Disciplines

5. Distribution by Journals (Figure 7)

No.	Journals	10 years number	Percentage	No.	Journals	3 years number	Percentage
1	ACADEMIC MEDICINE	2143	5.584	1	ACADEMIC MEDICINE	592	5.321
2	MEDICAL EDUCATION	1786	4.653	2	MEDICAL EDUCATION	419	3.766
3	MEDICAL TEACHER	1723	4.489	3	BMC MEDICAL EDUCATION	374	3.362
4	BMC MEDICAL EDUCATION	944	2.46	4	MEDICAL TEACHER	366	3.29
5	JOURNAL OF SURGICAL EDUCATION	871	2.269	5	JOURNAL OF SURGICAL EDUCATION	322	2.894
6	ACADEMIC PSYCHIATRY	762	1.985	6	ACADEMIC PSYCHIATRY	276	2.481
7	FAMILY MEDICINE	575	1.498	7	FAMILY MEDICINE	165	1.483
8	AMERICAN JOURNAL OF SURGERY	390	1.016	8	AMERICAN JOURNAL OF SURGERY	141	1.267
9	JOURNAL OF GENERAL INTERNAL MEDICINE	386	1.006	9	ADVANCES IN HEALTH SCIENCES EDUCATION	122	1.097
10	JAMA JOURNAL OF THE AMERICAN MEDICAL ASSOCIATION	376	0.98	10	JOURNAL OF THE AMERICAN COLLEGE OF RADIOLOGY	114	1.025

Figure 7　Distribution in Journals

Ⅱ. Research Fronts Analysis

1. High Frequent Keywords Analysis

Domain One

Education phase-General scope: Undergraduate education, Graduate education and Continuing education

From 2008-2017, the number of publications about Undergraduate education, Graduate education and Continuing education are 4622, 12627, and 3870, respectively. The publications on graduate education increased the fastest in the past five years with the largest number（Figure 8）.

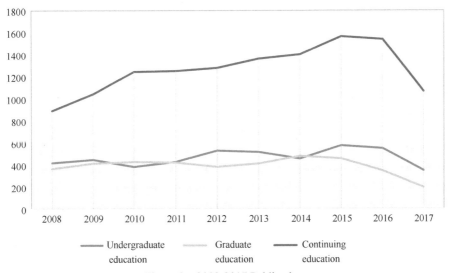

Figure 8   2008-2017 Publications

Note: Because the WOS database did not included all the 2017 publications, the number of medical education publications in this analysis is not intact. The missing part of 2017 publications will be included in the 2019 International Medical Education Research Fronts Report.

（1）Undergraduate education

Top 10 Keywords

1）Curriculum

2）Simulation（rate of last 3 years: 46%）

3）Assessment

4）PBL

5）E-learning（rate of last 3 years: 48%）

6）Clinical skills

7）Communication skills

8）Professionalism

9）Career choice

10）Active learning

Top 10 institutions

1）Univ Toronto

2）Maastricht Univ

3）Univ Calif San Francisco

4）Harvard Univ

5）Univ Michigan（rate of last 3 years: 43%）

6）Monash Univ

7）Univ British Columbia

8）Univ Sydney

9）Univ Illinois（rate of last 3 years: 47%）

10）Univ Calgary

（2）Graduate education

Top 10 Keywords

1）Simulation（rate of last 3 years: 44%）

2）Curriculum

3）Assessment

4）Patient safety

5）Communication skills

6）Teaching

7）Learning curve

8）Clinical competence

9）Primary care

10）Professionalism

Top 10 institutions

1）Harvard Univ

2）Univ Toronto

3）Univ Calif San Francisco

4）Mayo Clin

5）Univ Penn（rate of last 3 years: 40%）

6）Univ Michigan（rate of last 3 years: 39%）

7）Northwestern Univ

8）Univ Washington（rate of last 3 years: 41%）

9）Johns Hopkins Univ

10）Yale Univ

（3）Continuing education

Top 10 Keywords

1）Primary care

2）Simulation（rate of last 3 years: 37%）

3）Quality Improvement

4）Assessment

5）Learning curve

6）E-learning

7）Palliative care（rate of last 3 years: 31%）

8）Teaching

9）Knowledge translation

10）Patient safety

Top 10 institutions

1）Univ Toronto

2）Harvard Univ

3）Mayo Clin

4）Univ Calif San Francisco

5）Univ Washington（rate of last 3 years: 38%）

6）McMaster Univ

7）Univ Ottawa（rate of last 3 years: 41%）

8）Univ Calgary（rate of last 3 years: 38%）

9）Johns Hopkins Univ

10）McGill Univ

Domain Two

Study field-General scope: Curriculum, Educational Technology, Assessment, Teaching Methods, Education Management, Educational Policy（Figure 9）

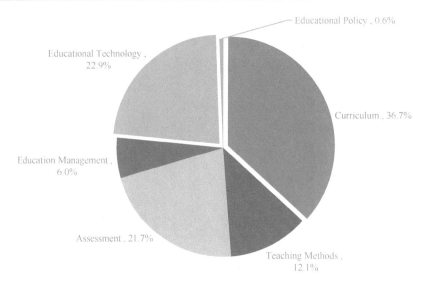

Figure 9 The Publication Distribution in Six Study Dields

（1）Curriculum

Top 10 Keywords

1）Competency-Based Education（rate of last 3 years: 38%）

2）Curriculum development

3）Milestones（rate of last 3 years: 70%）

4）Needs assessment

5）Feedback

6）Educational outcome

7）Simulation（rate of last 3 years: 57%）

8）Internship and residency

9）Learning（rate of last 3 years: 42%）

10）Pediatrics

Top 10 institutions

1）Univ Toronto（rate of last 3 years: 57%）

2）Harvard Univ（rate of last 3 years: 40%）

3）Univ Calif San Francisco（rate of last 3 years: 44%）

4）Yale Univ

5）Univ Massachusetts（rate of last 3 years: 71%）

6）Univ Ottawa（rate of last 3 years: 71%）

7) Univ Washington（rate of last 3 years: 57%）

8) Columbia Univ（rate of last 3 years: 67%）

9) Johns Hopkins Univ

10) Mayo Clin

（2）Educational Technology

Top 10 Keywords

1) Simulation（rate of last 3 years: 43%）

2) Training（rate of last 3 years: 41%）

3) E-learning

4) Virtual reality

5) Laparoscopy

6) Surgical education（rate of last 3 years: 43%）

7) Internet

8) Assessment

9) Social media（rate of last 3 years: 67%）

10) Virtual patients（rate of last 3 years: 40%）

Top 10 institutions

1) Univ Toronto

2) Harvard Univ

3) Mayo Clin

4) Univ London Imperial Coll Sci Technol & Med

5) Northwestern Univ

6) McGill Univ（rate of last 3 years: 51%）

7) Univ Calgary

8) Univ Ottawa（rate of last 3 years: 52%）

9) Johns Hopkins Univ

10) NYU

（3）Assessment

Top 10 Keywords

1) Feedback（rate of last 3 years: 46%）

2) Training

3) Simulation（rate of last 3 years: 44%）

4）Certification

5）Needs assessment

6）Accreditation

7）Milestones（rate of last 3 years: 68%）

8）AMEE Guide

9）Program evaluation

10）OSCE

Top 10 institutions

1）Univ Toronto（rate of last 3 years: 38%）

2）Harvard Univ

3）Maastricht Univ

4）Univ Calif San Francisco（rate of last 3 years: 42%）

5）Mayo Clin

6）Univ Ottawa（rate of last 3 years: 52%）

7）Univ Calif Los Angeles

8）Univ Michigan（rate of last 3 years: 53%）

9）Univ Washington

10）Johns Hopkins Univ（rate of last 3 years: 39%）

（4）Eaching Methods

Top 10 Keywords

1）Learning curve

2）Blended learning（rate of last 3 years: 42%）

3）Case study

4）Team-based learning

5）Simulation（rate of last 3 years: 56%）

6）E-learning

7）Experiential learning（rate of last 3 years: 47%）

8）Reflection

9）Standardized patients

10）Collaborative learning

Top 10 institutions

1）Maastricht Univ（rate of last 3 years: 46%）

2）Univ Toronto

3）Harvard Univ

4）Univ Calif San Francisco（rate of last 3 years: 39%）

5）Mayo Clin

6）Johns Hopkins Univ（rate of last 3 years: 54%）

7）Yale Univ（rate of last 3 years: 54%）

8）Brown Univ

9）Karolinska Inst

10）McGill Univ（rate of last 3 years: 70%）

（5）Education Management

Top 10 Keywords

1）Educational intervention（rate of last 3 years: 49%）

2）Workforce

3）Learning environment（rate of last 3 years: 40%）

4）School admission criteria（rate of last 3 years: 41%）

5）Specialty choice

6）Primary care

7）Educational impact

8）Continuing medical education（rate of last 3 years: 62%）

9）Educational needs/gaps

10）Guideline adherence

Top 10 institutions

1）Univ Toronto（rate of last 3 years: 67%）

2）Univ Michigan（rate of last 3 years: 73%）

3）Harvard Univ（rate of last 3 years: 50%）

4）Johns Hopkins Univ（rate of last 3 years: 60%）

5）Northwestern Univ（rate of last 3 years: 80%）

6）Mayo Clin

7）Univ Calif San Francisco

8）Univ N Carolina（rate of last 3 years: 44%）

9）Univ Washington

10）Univ Connecticut（rate of last 3 years: 62%）

（6）Educational Policy

Top 10 Keywords
1）Health services research
2）Rural health
3）Career choice
4）Career development
5）Emergency medicine
6）Family medicine
7）Graduate medical education
8）Primary care
9）Quality of care
10）Workforce

Top 10 institutions
1）Robert Graham Ctr（rate of last 3 years: 60%）
2）Harvard Univ（rate of last 3 years: 67%）
3）Univ Calif Los Angeles
4）Univ Penn
5）Univ Toronto
6）Assoc Amer Med Coll（rate of last 3 years: 100%）
7）Dartmouth Coll（rate of last 3 years: 50%）
8）Jichi Med Univ
9）Univ Calif San Francisco
10）Univ Virginia（rate of last 3 years: 100%）

Domain Three
CDCM-General scope: Clinical Skills & Patient Care, Core values & Professionalism, Preventive Disease & Health Promotion, Research Skills, Medical Knowledge & Lifelong Learning, Information & Management, Interpersonal & Communication Skills, Team Working Skills（Figure 10）

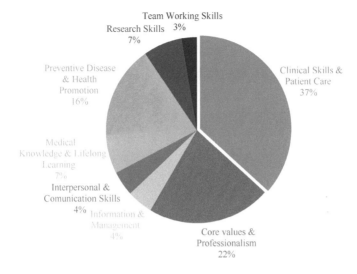

Figure 10   Publication Distribution in Eight Ability of Clinical Competency

（1）Clinical Skills & Patient Care

Top 10 Keywords

1）Primary care

2）Patient safety（rate of last 3 years: 39%）

3）Simulation（rate of last 3 years: 40%）

4）Clinical reasoning（rate of last 3 years: 37%）

5）Quality Improvement

6）Quality assurance

7）Assessment

8）Diagnosis

9）Physical examination

10）End-of–life care

Top 10 institutions

1）Univ Toronto

2）Harvard Univ

3）Univ Calif San Francisco

4）Univ Washington

5）Mayo Clin

6）Maastricht Univ

7）Johns Hopkins Univ

8）Yale Univ

9）Univ Calgary

10）Univ Penn

(2) Core values & Professionalism

Top 10 Keywords

1）Attitudes

2）Ethics（rate of last 3 years: 22%）

3）Workforce（rate of last 3 years: 32%）

4）Burnout（rate of last 3 years: 45%）

5）Empathy（rate of last 3 years: 43%）

6）Depression（rate of last 3 years: 39%）

7）Stress

8）Motivation（rate of last 3 years: 42%）

9）Training

10）Patient satisfaction

Top 10 institutions

1）Univ Toronto

2）Mayo Clin

3）Harvard Univ

4）Univ Calif San Francisco

5）Univ Michigan（rate of last 3 years: 52%）

6）Johns Hopkins Univ（rate of last 3 years: 41%）

7）Maastricht Univ（rate of last 3 years: 40%）

8）Massachusetts Gen Hosp（rate of last 3 years: 44%）

9）Univ Washington（rate of last 3 years: 44%）

10）Emory Univ（rate of last 3 years: 44%）

(3) Preventive Disease & Health Promotion

Top 10 Keywords

1）Quality improvement（rate of last 3 years: 47%）

2）Palliative care（rate of last 3 years: 39%）

3）Patient safety

4）Global health（rate of last 3 years: 49%）

5）Primary care

6）Curriculum（rate of last 3 years: 39%）

7）Graduate medical education（rate of last 3 years: 43%）

8）Older adults

9）Continuing medical education（rate of last 3 years: 48%）

10）Public health

Top 10 institutions

1）Univ Calif San Francisco（rate of last 3 years: 44%）

2）Harvard Univ

3）Univ Toronto（rate of last 3 years: 53%）

4）Univ Washington（rate of last 3 years: 63%）

5）Univ Calif Los Angeles（rate of last 3 years: 59%）

6）Johns Hopkins Univ（rate of last 3 years: 44%）

7）Univ Wisconsin

8）Emory Univ（rate of last 3 years: 43%）

9）Univ Michigan

10）Univ Minnesota（rate of last 3 years: 43%）

（4）Research Skills

Top 10 Keywords

1）Academic performance

2）Basic science

3）Training

4）Clinical research

5）Academic Productivity（rate of last 3 years: 43%）

6）Critical thinking

7）Academic Detailing

8）Innovation（rate of last 3 years: 47%）

9）Curriculum

10）Problem solving

Top 10 institutions

1）Univ Toronto

2）Harvard Univ

3）Mayo Clin（rate of last 3 years: 45%）

4）Univ Calif San Francisco

5）Univ British Columbia

6) Univ Ottawa

7) Univ Pittsburgh

8) Yale Univ (rate of last 3 years: 50%)

9) McMaster Univ

10) Dalhousie Univ

(5) Medical Knowledge & Lifelong Learning

Top 10 Keywords

1) Self-directed learning (rate of last 3 years: 40%)

2) Active learning

3) Knowledge translation

4) Attitudes

5) Interdisciplinary communication (rate of last 3 years: 43%)

6) Assessment

7) Continuing medical education

8) Undergraduate medical education

9) Evidence-based medicine

10) PBL

Top 10 institutions

1) Univ Toronto

2) McMaster Univ (rate of last 3 years: 40%)

3) Univ Laval

4) Univ Calgary

5) Univ Alberta

6) Univ Michigan

7) Dalhousie Univ

8) Harvard Univ (rate of last 3 years: 50%)

9) Mayo Clin (rate of last 3 years: 62%)

10) St Michaels Hosp

(6) Information & Management

Top 10 Keywords

1) Leadership

2) Health Policy

3) Resident duty hours

4) Quality management

5) Medical informatics

6) Information technology

7) Health manpower

8) Patient safety

9) Risk management

10) Continuing medical education

Top 10 institutions

1) Harvard Univ (rate of last 3 years: 46%)

2) Univ Toronto

3) Baylor Coll Med (rate of last 3 years: 43%)

4) Mayo Clin (rate of last 3 years: 43%)

5) Yale Univ

6) Univ Calif Los Angeles

7) Univ Michigan

8) Univ Penn

9) Univ Washington

10) Emory Univ

(7) Interpersonal & Communication Skills

Top 10 Keywords

1) Assessment

2) Training

3) Interprofessional collaboration (rate of last 3 years: 44%)

4) Patient-physician relationship (rate of last 3 years: 47%)

5) OSCE (rate of last 3 years: 42%)

6) Professionalism

7) Simulation

8) Residents

9) Medical students

10) Breaking bad news

Top 10 institutions

1) Univ Toronto

2) Catholic Univ Louvain

3) Harvard Univ (rate of last 3 years: 38%)

4）Univ Libre Bruxelles

5）Univ Liege

6）Duke Univ（rate of last 3 years: 50%）

7）Monash Univ

8）Radboud Univ Nijmegen

9）Univ Calif San Francisco（rate of last 3 years: 60%）

10）Free Univ Brussels

（8）Team Working Skills

Top 10 Keywords

1）Training

2）Simulation

3）Interprofessional education

4）Patient Safety

5）Leadership

6）Assessment

7）Surgery

8）Continuing medical education

9）Quality improvement

10）Faculty development

Top 10 institutions

1）Univ Toronto

2）Harvard Univ

3）Mayo Clin

4）Monash Univ

5）Univ Calif San Francisco（rate of last 3 years: 67%）

6）Univ London Imperial Coll Sci Technol & Med

7）Childrens Hosp Philadelphia

8）Karolinska Inst（rate of last 3 years: 50%）

9）Univ Sydney（rate of last 3 years: 50%）

10）Massachusetts Gen Hosp

Note: in the above 17 classifications, surgical education appeared in multiple categories. Combining with the publication distribution in discipline and journal, the results indicated that the surgical education obtained more attention and became the most important study field in comparison with other specialty education.

2. Reference Co-cited Clustering Analysis（Figure 11）

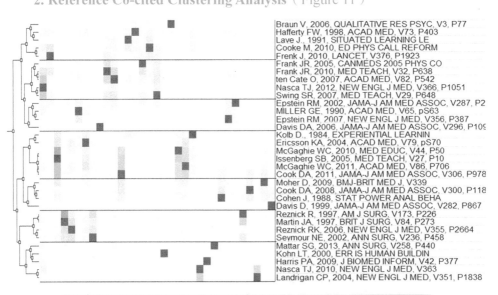

Braun V, 2006, QUALITATIVE RES PSYC, V3, P77
Hafferty FW, 1998, ACAD MED, V73, P403
Lave J, 1991, SITUATED LEARNING LE
Cooke M, 2010, ED PHYS CALL REFORM
Frenk J, 2010, LANCET, V376, P1923
Frank JR, 2005, CANMEDS 2005 PHYS CO
Frank JR, 2010, MED TEACH, V32, P638
ten Cate O, 2007, ACAD MED, V82, P542
Nasca TJ, 2012, NEW ENGL J MED, V366, P1051
Swing SR, 2007, MED TEACH, V29, P648
Epstein RM, 2002, JAMA-J AM MED ASSOC, V287, P2
MILLER GE, 1990, ACAD MED, V65, pS63
Epstein RM, 2007, NEW ENGL J MED, V356, P387
Davis DA, 2006, JAMA-J AM MED ASSOC, V296, P10S
Kolb D., 1984, EXPERIENTIAL LEARNIN
Ericsson KA, 2004, ACAD MED, V79, pS70
McGaghie WC, 2010, MED EDUC, V44, P50
Issenberg SB, 2005, MED TEACH, V27, P10
McGaghie WC, 2011, ACAD MED, V86, P706
Cook DA, 2011, JAMA-J AM MED ASSOC, V306, P978
Moher D, 2009, BMJ-BRIT MED J, V339
Cook DA, 2008, JAMA-J AM MED ASSOC, V300, P118
Cohen J, 1988, STAT POWER ANAL BEHA
Davis D, 1999, JAMA-J AM MED ASSOC, V282, P867
Reznick R, 1997, AM J SURG, V173, P226
Martin JA, 1997, BRIT J SURG, V84, P273
Reznick RK, 2006, NEW ENGL J MED, V355, P2664
Seymour NE, 2002, ANN SURG, V236, P458
Mattar SG, 2013, ANN SURG, V258, P440
Kohn LT, 2000, ERR IS HUMAN BUILDIN
Harris PA, 2009, J BIOMED INFORM, V42, P377
Nasca TJ, 2010, NEW ENGL J MED, V363
Landrigan CP, 2004, NEW ENGL J MED, V351, P1838

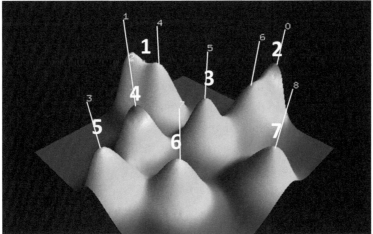

Figure 11　Reference Co-cited Clustering（2015-2017）

（1）The theory and practice of competency in medical education.

（2）Evaluation（Ability-oriented/evaluation methods）.

（3）Application of simulation enhancement technique in medical education.

（4）Teaching and Evaluation of Clinical Skills.

（5）Influence of working environment on the study and behavior of resident doctors and interned medical students.

（6）Interventional Study of medical education research and outcome evaluation.

（7）Others, including study environment, hidden curriculum, etc.

Conclusions

1. In the statistics of accumulative publications by countries, Brazil and China showed obvious advancement.

2. In the statistics of accumulative publications by institutions, Pennsylvania Uni. and the affiliated institutions showed great increase in last three years.

3. In the discipline statistics, medical education has witnessed more and more interdisciplinary research achievements in the past 3 years in surgery, cardiovascular system and mental illness.

4. In the journal statistics of accumulative publications, ADVANCES IN HEALTH SCIENCES EDUCATION and JOURNAL OF THE AMERICAN COLLEGE OF RADIOLOGY newly appeared in the top 10 journals in the last three years.

5. Among items of the three dimensions, post graduation education, clinical competence and patient care, core values and professionalism of physicians, education curriculum and educational technology have become the focus of attention.

6. In the frontiers of training, Simulation, Primary care, Professionalism and Patient safety have become the focus of attention.

7. In the frontier analysis of the competency research of clinicians, among the two themes, i.e. core values and physicians' professionalism/disease prevention and health promotion, more than half of the high frequency subject words have grown in the last 3 years, indicating that the two themes have been active recently.

8. In the frontier analysis of the research field, the cultivation concept of milestones and social media has been the most active focus of attention in the past 3 years. In addition, the competency and its related vocabulary appeared in many research fields and high-frequency subject words.

9. In the cluster analysis of citations, in addition to the theory and practice of competency in medical education and the application of simulation enhancement technology, the analysis results of high frequency subject words were further demonstrated. There were still learning environment, recessive courses and other contents in the analysis of the analysis.

Limitation

Both high frequency subject words statistics and citation clustering analysis techniques are based on high frequency and high cited data, which is better in catching the focus than covering all. However, in this study, the whole medical education research layout can be fully described through the classification and analysis of three dimensions.

Acknowledgement

Clarivate Group